MW01615391

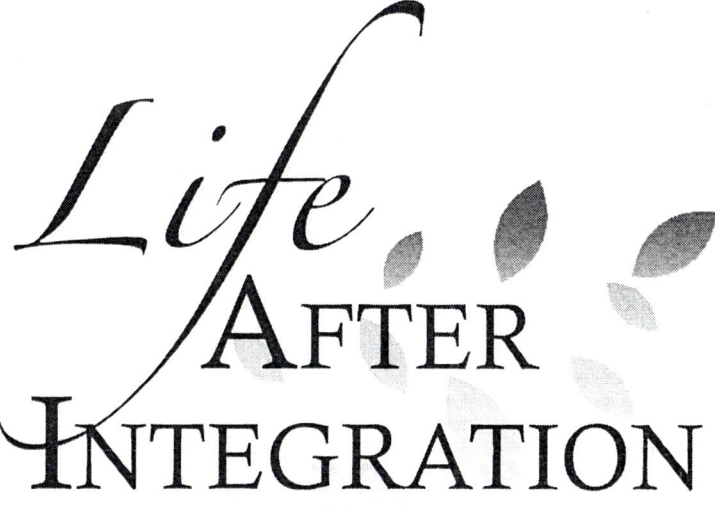

Life
AFTER
INTEGRATION

Much Love,
Teresa Liebscher

TERESA LIEBSCHER

TERESA LIEBSCHER
teresal@ibethel.org

TRANSFORMATION CENTER:
915 Twin View Blvd;
Redding, CA 96003
530-229-7909 ext 3001

Check out our website for further information on Sozo, the Sozo Network and Sozo training around the world.

www.bethelsozo.com

ISBN – 978-1-60445-100-9
Accent Digital Publishing • accentdigitalpublishing.com

Graphic Design and Book Formatting by Raina Pratt
rainapratt@gmail.com

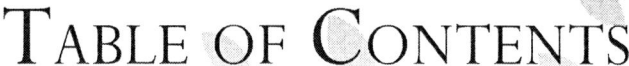

TABLE OF CONTENTS

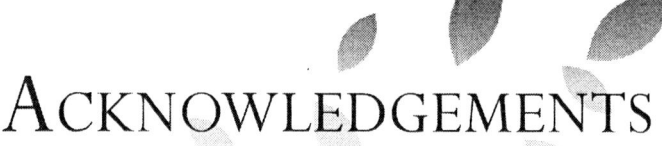

ACKNOWLEDGEMENTS

The first person I would like to say thank you to is my "partner in crime" Dawna De Silva. She took what I wrote in my very casual manner and helped turn it into something amazing. So thank you, Dawna, for being amazing and for supporting me.

Next is a group of people who cover the world (United States, Australia, Canada, England and Ireland) that "highly" encouraged me to write this book. You know who you are and thanks for the push, I think.

There is always that group of people who have their hands in the process of any project to see it through to the end. So not only a big thanks to Dawna, but also Sheryl, Sue and Raina.

Last but not least, to the family who has lived with me through this inherited life, what a journey.

Preface

I wrote this manuscript with the intent of bringing to light what could be expected for the client after completion of the Shabar Ministry or after being fully integrated through other inner healing ministry. This will be written from the point of view of both the person who has been either partially or fully healed as well as the journey of learning to live a "normal" life.

For the purpose of this writing, the definition of integration for the Shabar Ministry will be the process where all the broken places inside of the client have gone to be with Father God, Jesus, or the Holy Spirit. Simply put, complete integration would infer that the client will no longer have a connection to all of the "parts" or "protectors" that they have relied on throughout their life. Technically, the client will no longer see, hear, connect up to, or interact with what had previously been going on inside of them.

Therefore, an integrated person may feel empty inside, feel as if they have open space or their mind may seem quiet for the first time in their life. From this new perspective, this manuscript will look at the various markers along the journey from both the integrated person's viewpoint as well as their family and friends' perspective thus revealing the understanding of what is going on inside and outside of the newly integrated person.

Not all of these feelings, emotions, and consequences will occur with every client and their support groups. However, I believe that enough of them will occur as to warrant a sharing of this booklet, giving a head's up as to what to expect upon integration as well as what may follow in the years thereafter. A consideration for the integrated client should always be the possibility of losing all or part of what was in their current life: spouse, family, friends, ministry, job, etc. This aspect is very real and should be pondered by the client prior to the actual integration process. The "new you" may not be the same person as the one your husband or wife married, your friends enjoy, or your boss hired. To help demonstrate this examples of practical applications are included in the sections of this manuscript.

It should be noted that life after being healed might actually be harder for the client to walk through than the actual integration process itself. So as a healed, fully integrated person, who has gone before you, I speak hope to your journey into wholeness.

Teresa

1 MOMENT OF INTEGRATION

Clients have many different reactions to what has happened within them at the moment of integration. For sure, it will be the first time that they have a sense of being "clear minded." What they had lived and survived with for so many years will most likely no longer be there to help them process through future life situations. For some clients, they never considered the possibility of living life without their protectors and actually came seeking help not in getting "whole" but in managing their dysfunctions.

Several words clients have used to describe what they feel inside after integration is: empty, loss, an acknowledgement of empty space, or calm. The most common awareness is the inner silence, where previously it was an active, noisy place. In fact, this will most likely be the first time in the client's life that their brain has been silent and it can be quite unsettling for them.

A sense of disorientation or feeling "spacey" even to the point of being physically wobbly while standing or walking is also very common. It can feel like having sea legs while on land or a shifting center of gravity. For this reason, it is suggested that the client rest as much as possible after their Shabar sessions.

Eating well is also highly recommended. It should be noted that even though the client might not feel like they put forth a lot of effort in the session, the act of being integrated could be extremely exhausting for the client.

EXAMPLE:

I was sitting in the chair after the end of the session and my eyes were closed. All the parts that I had connected up to before were with Father God. I could not see, hear or connect up to them. I watched them interact and finally go be with Father God.

When the person ministering to me asked me how I felt or how it seemed inside, I realized that it was now totally different. I could not connect up to my protectors and there was no internal crisis going on. I no longer had the others shouting or arguing about things. This is when I realized it was quiet and calm. There was actually no noise at all going on inside and I felt spacey.

I opened my eyes. I started to look around and found that it seemed as if the room had changed. I knew that I had walked into this particular room but it now seemed more in focus, even the wall colors seemed brighter.

The minister was watching me and asked if I felt disoriented and I realized this was an accurate word for how I felt. That was a good word for it. Yes, I was definitely disoriented, and tired, but also excited. It was a very strange set of emotions.

2 LEAVING THE SESSION

After the integration process, the person will most likely experience a type of sensory overload. This will be the first time the client will have looked out of "one set of eyes" instead of seeing through several lenses at once. The world will therefore look, feel and be sensed differently than before the session. This could cause the client to either respond much slower or even quicker to situations or issues they encounter. It will be like looking at the world and all that is in it for the first time, like never having seen these things before. And, in reality, it is true. Before their session, life had been filtered through a completely different set of lenses.

From this point on, the client will have to learn how to live life without their prior inner parts/protectors. It can be a very vulnerable time for the newly integrated person while they have to relearn how to handle every day situations of communication and conflict. Many will have to learn how to live with their mind quiet for the first time. This can be very unnerving for the newly integrated person and they will need to give themselves grace in learning how to live without the constant noise that has been with them all their lives. Many clients will need to have outside sources – TV, radio, music – playing so as not to be completely disoriented by this new silence.

Other clients may actually begin to grieve the loss of these internal voices as though they lost a good friend.

This is a very good time to begin training the client how to connect to Father God, Jesus, and the Holy Spirit so that when they find themselves in now unfamiliar situations, they will be able to hear what He suggests they should do.

EXAMPLE:

As I was walking out of the office after the integration, I was trying to find the other parts. Looking to them to come and help me deal with the disorientation going on inside of me. The parts, however, were not there, no longer vying for attention, demeaning their own actions or arguing about my current situation.

The person ministering to me had mentioned that it would be like seeing out of one set of eyes instead of several at the same time, as I had grown accustomed to. He told me to begin looking at the objects around me as I made my way to the car. When I looked up at the trees, it actually seemed like each leaf was so much clearer, sharper than I had noticed before. I have had people say when they got glasses they could even see the points of pine needles at the tops of the trees. It was like that sharper, clearer, and distinct.

There was an awareness of my surroundings, as I had never felt before. It seemed like there was more space around me, physically and in the spiritual realm. I started feeling overwhelmed with what was going on and feeling vulnerable with no place to hide. I was on sensory overload and there wasn't any place left inside for me to run away to.

Someone started to talk to me and I realized that the sounds around me seemed distorted, louder and strange, the person even looked different than before.

It is noteworthy to mention here that a newly integrated person can re-fracture if he is not able to cope with this new level of input, perception and comprehension of the world around him/her. Grace should be extended to the client if this is the option he chooses. Although fractured people aren't sure how they created the parts in the first place, if feeling overwhelmed or unprotected, new parts may come into play. Once the client realizes what has occurred, the client can use the Shabar tools on himself/herself to integrate these newly created parts.

EXAMPLE:

> As I lived each day after the integration, situations that I had handled numerous times before occurred, but now I did not know how to respond to them. It was like these common occurrences were coming my way for the first time. I was unsure of what I should do, how I should handle each situation, or what was the proper way to behave. In fact, these common situations were now new to me because I no longer had the parts inside responding. Most of the time, I did not do the socially correct thing that people of my age were expected to do.

In dealing with these situations, it is possible that the newly integrated person becomes so overwhelmed that they shut down in this stressful moment and a new protector/part of them comes forth to help

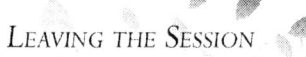

them cope with the overload. Several days or weeks later, the client may realize that this new part was created. If the client can begin gathering useful communication skills and/or hear and accept God's truth about the situation, then the new part will no longer be needed and the client can use his Shabar tools to reintegrate this new part.

3 FRIENDS, FAMILY & CHURCH FAMILY

Life after integration is stepping into an inherited life, that the integrated person did not choose. Others inside created this life. These parts/protectors are the ones that have connected socially with those around them. The newly integrated person steps back into life with all of these people around who have a connection to the "old self" but the new self who now stands in front of them may have a completely changed personality with different desires, behaviors, and even needs. This can be confusing and unsettling to both the client and those they are in relationship with.

The integrated client will not present as the same person they were prior to integrations: the spouse is no longer the same person the spouse met and married, the parent is no longer the parent the children grew up with, he/she is no longer the friend the family and friends have learned to tolerate or enjoy. Family and friends will need to decide if they would even like to reconnect with the newly integrated person. It can be quite a learning curve for all involved.

So what if all these people do not like the newly integrated spouse/parent/friend? What if they don't want this new connection? What if they don't want to put in the time to learn new healthy ways of reconnecting to each other? And what if the family and friends do not want to look at themselves now and see how they contributed and partnered with the client's previous behaviors?

The client and spouse will most likely need marriage counseling to deal with these issues that were present in the past but never properly addressed. Added stress in the marriage is common during this time of relearning and if the spouse is willing, he/she will need to understand and work with the client to rebuild a new healthy relationship. Children of a newly integrated person may get very angry with this "new" parent who no longer allows the children to manipulate and direct what happens within the family unit. Confusion may become part of the atmosphere that the family will need to deal with as the newly integrated parent learns how to set proper boundaries within the home.

A friend may be used to taking care of the integrated person and once the client becomes whole, the role of caretaking is no longer needed this will cause confusion and strain on a friendship based solely on care giving. In many cases, the caregiver actually becomes angry with the newly integrated person because they are no longer needed in their life.

Each party will either need to make new healthy connections or they will simply begin to disconnect, ultimately abandoning the newly integrated person. This is a very real cost of integration to the client.

Parents or other family members of the integrated person as well may also be upset with the new persona that is now disrupting the family with their different opinions, likes, and boundaries. No longer needing to "keep the peace" can cause explosive family dynamics either by the family members blowing up or the client learning now how to deal with negative emotions of anger, fear, jealousy, etc. Many times, these new family dynamics cause others in the family to have to recognize themselves as part of the problem, and many people would rather continue to blame the client instead of owning their own sins. Some family members will actually try to pull the client back into unhealthy family patterns so that they do not have to look at themselves and their own need to change. It will be important for the newly integrated person to understand this dynamic and be ready to have a healthy approach to resisting falling back into prior unhealthy patterns.

Many times, family members will use new outbursts of negative emotion displayed by the newly integrated person as a sign that the client is not actually healed, rather than allowing the client to learn proper ways to handle these newly acquired emotions. These changed behaviors can be very confusing and frustrating to family members who have adjusted over the years to the prior "normal" dysfunction.

EXAMPLE:

> During dinner at a restaurant, my spouse started talking about how he has really not seen much difference in me after my being integrated. He said he doesn't see me handling situations any differently. I began to get mad and tune him out because I know that I have been handling situations in a different way than I did two or six months ago. I internally feel the anger differently than before. I am not losing control or running away from daily reality. I agree that I am probably not yet handling my life situations as well as other healthy individuals but I am working to do so. So his statements are confusing to me. Am I in denial? Am I truly whole?

4 LIVING LIFE, OLD & NEW TOOLS

The integration process has removed all of the old tools used by the parts/protectors to handle reality. Life feels and looks different even when those around the client may not see the changes. The client may even be dealing with the possibility of losing all or part of their prior life connections: spouse, family, friends, ministry, job, etc.

Even though the client has been in their life situations many times before, they have never encountered these stressors as a whole person. Thus, he/she will be at a loss as to how to cope with these possible life issues and new tools will need to be acquired by the client in order to properly handle them. These tools should have been learned in early childhood but are still foreign to the newly integrated person. Society as a whole has a difficult time in allowing an adult to learn the social skills they should already have mastered. Grace is given to little children to learn how to have social and relational skills, but seldom do we give the same grace to a newly integrated person learning these new skills.

There are numerous places to learn the skills the client is now lacking: college, books, counseling, mentoring, cell & home groups, relationships with people and attending church and group functions.

Attending conferences and seminars for developing such ministry and interpersonal skills will be very helpful to the newly integrated person. Going back to school and increasing writing and reading skills can actually be quite liberating to the newly whole person.

It will be mostly by trial and error that the newly integrated person begins to acquire such skills since it isn't until life situations present themselves that the client realizes skills are actually missing. The client will most likely make quite a few mistakes along the way. Mistakes in social interactions, communication, and interpersonal skills are a sign of integration and should therefore be seen as an symbol that total integration has occurred rather than just a loss of proper etiquette.

Discovering new tools will mean that the client will have to now deal with life realities – something that they deferred to in the past to their protectors/parts. Situations that were once easily handled will now be uncomfortable and possibly overwhelming. It is in these situations that the client will realize that they are missing the proper "tools" society expects them to already have. As these situations present themselves, the newly integrated person will need to seek out where to learn the skills needed and will also need to release grace to themselves while doing so. The counselor should not be looking for correct reactions to life situations but rather that the client is not re-fracturing or "going away". Even meltdowns can therefore be interpreted as proof that the client is progressing.

It will take time for the client to learn to find the balance of handling each situation that will be faced. Commonly the newly integrated person will swing from one side of emotions to the other while learning how to properly handle life. It will take time to learn how to properly present himself/herself in each new situation.

EXAMPLE:

Since I have been healed, my trips to the dentist are so different than before my healing process. Before integration, I would be in tears to even enter the dental lobby. Since then, I have gone a few times for teeth cleanings and amazingly I didn't have any tears.

One particular trip I needed a crown, which meant needles! I was thinking, "I'll be fine. I have been doing so well." I was a bit nervous but no tears came as I entered the lobby and still no tears as I was led to the chair. Teary eyes welled up however as the needle was used to numb my cheek area and I realized that I was looking for a part to come forth and rescue me from my current ordeal. No one come forth and I didn't quite know what to do. I realized that I was going to need to hook up to the Holy Spirit to teach me a new tool in order to handle these types of situations.

In other circumstances where I have recognized my lack of appropriate skills, I took classes and read books regarding a particular situation so I could watch how others handled them.

This can be potentially embarrassing to the client if they feel they are caught unaware of how to handle themselves and it is helpful if their support group would extend to them grace, support them and even point them to safe places to learn the relationship skills they are missing.

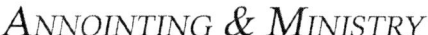

ANNOINTING & MINISTRY

There may be a need to relearn the aspects of one's abilities and giftings in connection to the ministry or church activities involved with prior to integration. Usually there is no loss of abilities or giftings but since the integrated person is looking at life and situations from a different set of eyes, these abilities and giftings will be viewed or processed now differently. Because a fractured person lives in a heightened state of fear, they may have seemed to have a high level of discernment prior to integration which no longer functions in quite the same manner.

EXAMPLE:

> I have always been able to know what is going on around me without having to even think about it. I would know before interacting with people who was safe and what their motives were. Now after integration, this awareness dramatically changed. The markers I used to sum up situations quickly had morphed and I was unsure of how to read people now. It was a new learning curve in how to figure out

not only what was going on but how I would respond once I figured it out.

My connection with Father God, Jesus and the Holy Spirit was also different. Up to and through my healing process, I was going between being really mad at God and confused about each of their functions in my life. Now, my closer, clearer connection to God was both over-whelming and exciting. I needed to learn how to redirect my senses to also deal with the spiritual realm.

This is because the information that had been collected from the Godhead and the spiritual realm prior to integration was coming from several directions at once. The client will now need to learn how to discern from this new healed, focused place and minister confidently from there.

PERSONAL CHANGES

Personal changes will undoubtedly occur. A new taste in the style of clothing, accessories, food, and arrangement of the home furnishings will be experienced because in reality someone other than the newly integrated person had chosen the previous styles through many sets of likes and dislikes. Before integration one type of food may have been especially enjoyed and now may not be liked at all. On the flip side, foods that would never have been tried before now may be eaten and surprisingly enjoyed.

Personal changes often occur about every six months as the person experiments and discovers these newly acquired tastes and styles of clothing, decorations and food. This usually lasts about two years. After this time, the changes slow down until they finally become pretty well set for the client.

It is important in the healing process therefore to go ahead and experiment with tastes and colors. Try different styles and colors of clothing, new flavors of foods, new genres of entertainment (books, movies, TV shows) that would not have been tried prior to integration. Don't worry about getting stuck with certain styles you won't like in the future. Other than tattoos, new expressions of tastes should not be seen as permanent during this trial phase towards wholeness.

EXAMPLE:

As the first week was continuing after the integration, I was looking at my clothes in the closet and there were three different styles and sizes that I had chosen and I realized I really didn't like any of them. As I stood and stared at the clothes, I realized, I didn't really know what style I would actually like. Up to now, I had worn mostly browns and blacks (so I could hide) and none of them would have been considered trendy.

Food was another adventure for me. Up to the time of the integration, thinking about tasting food I was not sure I would like would physically make me ill. Now I was interested in what other foods tasted like and I wanted to try some new foods. At the same time, I would eat food that I had previously liked only to find that I no longer enjoyed them.

PHYSICAL HEALING

Fractured people usually have some kind of physical issue. After the integration, the physical issues will also begin to heal. Once the body realizes that the integrated person will deal with reality in a healthy manner and it (the body) will no longer have to fight to deal with the entire crisis, it will begin to rest properly, deal with stress properly, and begin to heal and be able to maintain a healthy immune system. Our bodies are so interconnected with our belief systems that it has been common among our clients to have an average of ninety percent of all prior physical issues no longer be present within two years of integration.

EXAMPLE:

> I had several physical issues for as long as I can remember. Some of them the doctors know about and some no one else but me knew of. One of those physical issues had me in the doctor's office or emergency room several times a year. I would be sick from one to four months each time with bronchitis and sometimes in bed for several weeks at a time. About a year after the integration, I realized I had not dealt with bronchitis in several months, had not seen the doctor, or been to the hospital for treatment. I then begun to check

out my other physical issues and realized that I was either free of them or about 85% better with each one.

5 RELATIONSHIP WITH GODHEAD

Up to this point, most fractured people's connection with the Godhead has been in constant conflict. Now there is an opportunity to develop a healthy intimate relationship with each member of the Godhead - an opportunity to learn about the true nature and character of Father God, Jesus, and the Holy Spirit. In this new, unknown territory that the integrated person is journeying through, making mistakes, learning new tools, and applying new tools, there is a need to find out what God will do. To discover if God will come through for him/her and protect him/her and whether He will "back" the decisions the now whole person has begun to make.

As life is being lived and experimented with, there will be a need to lean on this new developing relationship with God. It is important to remember what each member of the Godhead promised him/her during the integration process.

EXAMPLE:

> Before the integration process, I was never sure if what I was hearing, seeing or feeling was really from God or from one of my inner voices. I thought Father God was upset or

43

mad at me and since He didn't really like me, he had no reason to pay attention to me, or my prayers. On top of this, I was not reacting or having the same connections with God as the people in church around me. People began telling me that everything I was dealing with was my own imagination and that too confused me further with whose voice I was truly hearing or responding to.

After the integration, all of this was changed. I could tell now that what I had heard or seen for myself was God or me. I could feel God for the first time and I could believe what He was telling me.

The ability to perceive God now from a place of single mindedness is a huge step in the integrated persons healing process.

6 RELATIONSHIP WITH FAMILY & FRIENDS

Family and friends may have a difficult time adjusting to the differences the newly integrated person displays in tastes, moods, and character. They may have to deal with a whirlwind of changes in the client just as the client has to handle the changes within himself/herself. The view for the family and friends, however, will come from an outside perspective that differs from that of the client himself/herself and what the client may be perceiving as appropriately handled situations may in fact be triggering family and friends into responding negatively to these new changes.

Family and friends have grown accustomed to responding in a particular way to the client and vice versa. Now, a different, foreign response is coming at them from the client. Most family and friends will not know how to respond instantly to the changes coming from the client. It is very common, therefore, for family and friends to also seek help to learn how to set and hold onto new boundaries and communicate properly with the client.

The newly integrated person's physical look may even be different. The family/friend's patterns of living life will not have changed as the integrated person's patterns will have changed. They will continue to live life just like before, but the old family patterns may not work well for the newly integrated person because he/she is so completely different. This usually causes disruptions in the family and friend's dynamics.

The client should release understanding and grace to the family and friends until they are able to see the client as truly healed and changed. This will take time and even more time will be needed for all the changes to come across as positive to the family and friends. When negative emotions arise from a newly integrated person who had always been compliant in the past, the family and friends may actually feel like the client has regressed when he/she is really just trying to find new, proper responses. Time following integration is usually harder on the client and family relationships than pre-integration even though healthy boundaries and lifestyles are now being formed and followed.

It may be helpful for the client to communicate with a spouse and a couple of close friends about what has taken place during the process of integration. They may be able to help the client set up signs or key words that they could say or show during communication with others, that would let the client know whether their response to others is appropriate or out of bounds. This will also benefit the spouse and friends who will realize that the newly integrated person is not running away but is actually having a hard time dealing with new found emotions and situations.

The time of experimenting may be strange for the family and friends as well as the client and again grace will be a key to success for the whole family unit. The newly integrated person will not be used to trying new things or actually having an opinion and therefore will not know what to do when their opinions are not welcomed. It will take a great commitment from both parties to allow mistakes and for the client to not automatically spiral downward when clashes occur.

Family and friends may be disoriented when there is an expectation of one way to handle situations. Many times, as the newly integrated person learns and applies healthy tools to family dynamics, the relatives are caught off balance and are forced to learn healthy tools themselves. It should be noted that not all of the family and friend's reactions to the client are healthy or proper. The client will need to learn how to handle family and friends responses when they are not appropriate, without assuming fault for the dysfunction.

EXAMPLE:

> When my friends starting realizing that something was different about me, they had various reactions. Some were confused, some were upset, some were even mad. Some have not talked to me since. My friends did not know how to handle the new me. They did not know how to interact with me while I was learning the new tools I needed in order to handle social interactions and confrontations appropriately.

> One day one of my friends and I were talking about how different I was and how our relationship had changed. In the past, I seemed to always need her advice before I could make up my mind regarding decisions. Now I was not even asking her about my life needs and this was unsettling for her. She realized she was also a bit mad at me. She was so use to her advisory role in my life she was not sure she liked not advising me.

One by one, many of my friends began to distance themselves from me until very few of my pre-integration friends remained by my side. I did, however, have some who decided to hang with the new me. It was not always easy on them since they had to deal with the tension of my learning how to use new tools, process the ups and downs of my newly expressed emotions, trying to find my new foundation and even deciding the proper boundaries in my life. One of my friends described my after years of this process as "watching me grow from a two year old to a sixty year old woman all in a span of five years."

7 RELATIONSHIP WITH THE CHURCH

For the integrated person's church, the reactions can be the same as with family and friends. Church members and Co-workers will expect a certain reaction from the client as dictated by past experiences. Even though healing has occurred and the client has appropriated proper new tools, the church may be cautious towards the client in serving or ministering in the church. Grace and understanding need to be released by the client as the church learns to trust the new person before them.

The church may, if the integrated person has been doing ministry, ask him/her to step down from ministry for a time to see if the healing process has actually been effective and to make sure the client handles situations appropriately. This should not be seen as an offensive move toward the client but an understandable response of the church leadership while the integrated person becomes whole.

EXAMPLE:

> At the time of my healing process, I was involved in a ministry at my church. The leader of the ministry knew about the healing process. The ministry leader decided that

it might be good idea if I was not involved in ministry at this time. The leadership was unsure of how the integration process would affect my ability to minister. They were also wary of the changes they were observing. There was also concern about how I was handling this new place in life and how I was wielding the new tools I was learning.

At first I was confused, hurt and mad. Not only were my family and friends pulling away from me but also now the church was doing the same. I had thought that being in ministry would actually speed up my new connection to God. However, as I processed this perceived rejection by the church leadership, I realized that I had a place with Father God to process this pain and submit my confusion, hurt and anger to Him.

8 THE JOURNEY AFTERWARDS

R ight after I was integrated I had a picture of what life was going to be for me, I saw these really big wooden doors. They felt 20 feet tall, 10 feet deep. Someone opened them up just enough for a hand to push me through them. As soon as I was on the other side, the doors were closed and I was unable to turn around and go back through them. As I stood there, with my back to the doors, I looked out in front of me and saw nothing but dirt and sand. There were no plants, no trees, no buildings, no landscapes, nothing. Then I heard (sensed maybe) that this was now my life. I could do what I wanted. I was the one choosing the planting materials, and building the buildings. I could see something very far off in the distance but I could not see or figure out what it was. There was no sense that I would be alone in this journey. Even there I had to accept that this empty landscape was my life. I was not a happy person. I wanted to turn away and go back through the doors, but I could not and to be honest I was very mad I could not go back through the doors.

Now that you have read all about the life after integration, about how life is going to be changed for the newly integrated person, let me talk about the amazing journey you are about to go on or you have already started. This will be from the viewpoint of a fully integrated person. For those of you who have had some integration but realized there may or could still be parts/protectors still there, please know there is light at the end of the tunnel for you.

This life afterwards has been an amazing journey for me, which I would not give up even knowing how hard it has been. It will be a journey until the very end. For I am sure I will continue to have lots of opportunities to learn new healthy tools and continue to refine those tools to deal with life situations.

The first aspect of this amazing journey is my relationship with each member of the Godhead. To learn about the nature and character of the Godhead and how They each wish to interact with me and my life. I am watching Them care and protect me like I have never known in my life. I watch Them teach me about life and about the tools that are needed to deal with people and situations in life. It has not been easy, at times I don't like what I am being taught or what is expected of me.

The first aspect of the journey leads to the second:

how to deal with life and people. Once I was able to trust each member of the Godhead, I could learn to connect and properly interact with people. Proper interaction with people aids proper dealing with the life situations that will come. Interaction with people and life dynamics give endless opportunity to learn and develop knowledge and healthy interacting tools. In this opportunity I get to decide if I am going to connect up with the Godhead, decide which tool I am going to use with the people and/or situations. Will I use one of the new tools I have learned or will I decide to use an unhealthy, old tool in an uncomfortable situation?

Along the way I have had my ups and downs. I have not always used the tools properly or even at the right times. I have availed myself of the Godhead and at times not wanted to listen to Them or use the directions They gave me.

Yet through it all, this journey has been fun, this is the most solid I have ever felt in my life. I may get afraid, worried, feel rejected, I might struggle with the life I inherited but I now know I don't have to go away inside to deal with what is being handed to me. I can stay present no matter what.

Now to go back to the picture I talked about at the beginning of this chapter, the undeveloped landscape has changed so much as I have gone through my journey. When I go back and visit that picture, there is so much going on, a mature garden, buildings, sounds, colors, life. Are there areas in my garden that need work and don't look as well as they should, yes of course! Yet part of the healthy journey is to be able to acknowledge them and work on a plan to improve those areas. I can still see the doors, I have no desire to journey back to them. At times it might be nice to go revisit what was built at the beginning of my journey, but I cannot change anything so I just keep focused on the present and enjoy what is developed around me now.

We all have our landscapes that are unknown territory and items we are building around us. Now as a healed person, you get to choose what you are going to do with your landscape, and not let what is inside of you control your decisions.

This journey of integration is not a sprint, it is a marathon. There will be mistakes made and messes to clean up but that doesn't mean that you still have parts/protectors. It is an opportunity to learn new tools to deal with the realities of life. It takes time and you must give yourself grace for each aspect of your journey.

The cost of the integration process can be high, but the benefits are worth it. It is a decision you will have to make for yourself. This is your life, your choices and your ability to relate with other people. Yet let me invite you into an amazing journey with Father God, Jesus, Holy Spirit, people and life.